Workout Routines for Women

How to Get Fit By Doing Aerobic Exercises

By: Jana Duncan

9781630225674

I0413984

TABLE OF CONTENTS

Jana Duncan
Publishers Notes

Speedy Publishing LLC

40 E. Main St., #1156

Newark, DE 19711

www.speedypublishing.co

Cover Artwork: 24 Hr. Designs Ltd.

Editing: Speedy Publishing LLC

Book design: Speedy Publishing LLC

ISBN: 9781630225674

This is a reprint book.

DISCLAIMER

This publication is intended to provide helpful and informative material. It is not intended to diagnose, treat, cure, or prevent any health problem or condition, nor is intended to replace the advice of a physician. No action should be taken solely on the contents of this book. Always consult your physician or qualified health-care professional on any matters regarding your health and before adopting any suggestions in this book or drawing inferences from it.

The author and publisher specifically disclaim all responsibility for any liability, loss or risk, personal or otherwise, which is incurred as a consequence, directly or indirectly, from the use or application of any contents of this book.

Any and all product names referenced within this book are the trademarks of their respective owners. None of these owners have sponsored, authorized, endorsed, or approved this book.

Always read all information provided by the manufacturers' product labels before using their products. The author and publisher are not responsible for claims made by manufacturers.

DEDICATION

To Sheila - I had you in mind for these routines.

CHAPTER 1- BENEFITS OF AEROBIC EXERCISE

An interesting fact about aerobics is that the word aerobics was created by the founder of the Cooper Institutes founder Kenneth H. Cooper, M.D., a sports exercise physiologist.

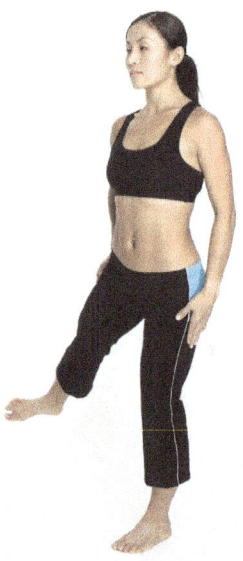

We are always reminded that exercise could do wonders for the body. Aerobics, a kind of exercise which helps your body use more oxygen while maintaining your target heart rate; can definitely help a person live longer and healthier. There are studies showing that 30 minutes of aerobics every day would benefit the body a lot.

Performing regular aerobic exercises would gradually make the heart larger. A bigger and larger heart would be able to provide more oxygenated blood which can be used by the muscles. This could also mean more energy whether for longer or shorter periods of exercise or physical activities.

Jana Duncan
Weight loss

Aerobics and any kind of physical activity could surely help control and reduce weight. It is most successful when combined with a healthy diet. Including physical activity and exercise with your daily routine will surely help you achieve better built, healthy lifestyle and increase in energy. Aerobics would help your body burn the calories consumed and prevent them from becoming accumulated fats.

Stronger Resistance against Sickness

Aerobics can boost the body's immune system. This would prevent illnesses like colds and flu from happening. It could also help the body manage existing health problems like high blood pressure and blood sugar. Excessive weight and obesity could cause serious health problems like diabetes, heart disease and stroke. Aerobics could help in reducing the risks of these diseases. This kind of exercise could help in clearing the arteries of the heart from bad cholesterol.

• Elderly Benefits

Aging could have different effects on the body and exercise could help you deal with these changes. It could help your body become stronger and more mobile when you grow old. Common problems of the elderly would be flexibility and mobility. Aerobics and maintaining other forms of exercise even when older would help reduce these problems.

• Increase in Stamina and Energy

Contrary to what some people think, aerobics and exercise wouldn't leave you breathless and less energetic. It could boost your stamina and energy. Continuous and regular exercise could result to muscle development and increase in body endurance. Aside from that, aerobics could also reduce fatigue and decrease shortness of breath. Aerobics could help the body achieve better sleep at night, making the person more energetic and fresh the next day.

• Promote Better Mental Health

Exercise does not only calm and help the body; it could also help in boosting a mood of a person. Achieving better health and physical results through aerobics could increase self-esteem and self-confidence. It is even used to reduce stress, anxiety and depression.

Aerobics have numerous benefits. In fact, some would say that aside from physical and mental benefits, aerobics could also help in improving sexual performance. There are also different types of aerobic exercises which could capture the interest of people with different ages and characteristics.

However, aerobics may not be safe for everybody. Those with certain illnesses and those that are pregnant should take necessary precautions when performing aerobic exercises. Before trying any aerobic routine, it is important to consult with a doctor first especially if you have an existing or past medical condition.

CHAPTER 2- DIFFERENT TYPES OF AEROBIC EXERCISES

The term aerobics is coined from the word aerobic which means "with oxygen."

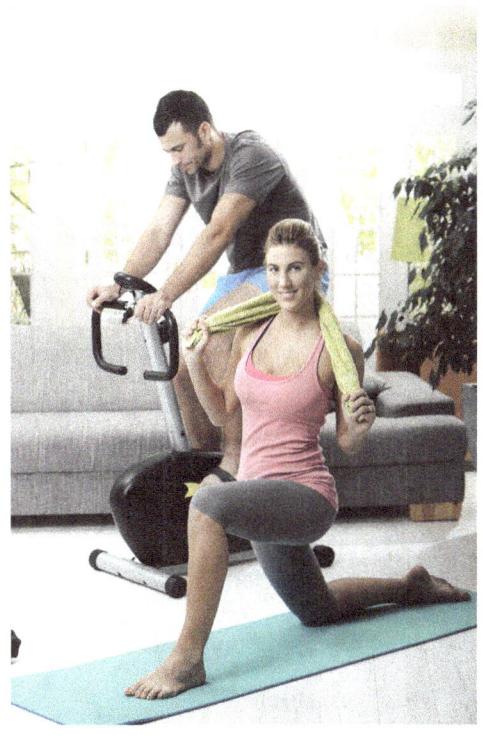

Aerobics is one of the most popular types of exercises in the market. Its use of music, dance, equipment and other facilities have contributed to its popularity. Aerobic exercises are workouts that intend to increase the heart rate for a period of time. This would cause the body to have higher intake of oxygen which would result into better blood circulation, weight loss, faster calorie and fat burning.

Other physical activities can also be considered as aerobic workouts, like swimming, running, walking, jogging, and cycling. An aerobic exercise would start with a 5 to 10 minutes of warm-up stretching and exercises. After the warming-up, the routine proper would follow, lasting for about 20 to 30 minutes. The last part of the workout will be the cooling-down process.

There are different types of aerobic exercises for different levels of individuals. Skill, health and comfort are things to be considered when choosing what type of aerobic exercise would fit with the individual's needs and abilities. Some of the types are:

• **Low-Impact Aerobics**

As the name implies, low-impact exercises don't include activities which could harm the bones and joints like jumping and bouncing. Exercises performed had lower intensity, thus reducing the risks of injuries and leg overuse. In this exercise, one or both feet should always be in contact with the ground.

With low-impact routine, you do not start with a high note. An individual could start performing the exercises on a slower rate and gradually increase its intensity. Low-impact aerobics is ideal for seniors, obese and overweight individuals and of course, pregnant women.

• **High Impact Aerobics**

High impact aerobic exercises use different movements. It could include jumping, turning, shuffling, doubling, etc. This kind of workout intends to develop the abdominal area, calf, and also the cardiovascular system. If an individual is agile and active prior to working out, then high-impact aerobics may be the best option. But for beginners, slower and low-impact exercises is recommended first. When the individual is already comfortable with this low-impact level, then it would be safe to proceed with the second level. Keep in mind that doctor's discretion is always important.

• Step Aerobics

Step aerobics uses step benches for working out. This kind of aerobics is actually low in impact. There are studies showing that step aerobics can help a person reduce weight, given the fact that its impact is only half of the impact used when riding a bike at home. Overall, this process or workout is dedicated for the development of the lower body.

• Aerobic Kickboxing

It is also called cardio boxing. This is one of the most effective workouts for losing weight. Although, aerobic kickboxing is tiring, its effects on the body are great. It could definitely help in building more energy and longer stamina. It is also called cardioboxing and can burn about 800 calories in an hour.

• Water Aerobics

Another low-impact exercise but delivers huge results, whether it is for weight loss or improving over-all health. Water aerobics, according to experts, burns calories faster compared with land-exercises because of the water's resistance.

CHAPTER 3- WADING IN WATER AEROBICS

Swimming is one of the top five aerobic exercise options.

Physical activities like walking, running, dancing and swimming can be considered aerobics. Aerobics are exercises which increase the heart rate and at the same time pump more oxygen into the blood vessels. There are different kinds of aerobic exercises which can be defined based on the equipment used in the workout program. Water aerobic workout is an example of an aerobic workout.

Water aerobics or aqua aerobics can also be referred to as waterobics. This kind of workout is usually performed in a swimming pool with waist-deep water. It could be in an indoor or outdoor pool, with water temperature of 82º F to 86º F. Come to think of it, the most common form of waterobics is swimming. Water aerobics would focus on building body strength, flexibility, balance and providing a cardiovascular workout. It's one session usually lasts for about 40 to 50 minutes.

Just like any other aerobic workout, there is a five-minute warm-up and would end with five-minute cool-down. There could be floatation devices provided to the participants if the water is deep. Kickboards and water barbells are also provided to help participants afloat or can be used for exercises. Water weights and floating belts are also used to increase water resistance. Music is used during workout sessions.

When kicking off with waterobics, the most basic thing that you need is your swimsuit. There are some participants who would also use a swimming cap to keep the hair out of the face and special aqua shoes. These special shoes can support you ankles and also prevent your feet from slipping. They would also serve as protection against cuts and scrapes.

There are numerous benefits from including water aerobics in your lifestyle.

• Since water provides buoyancy and support to the body, there is less risk of bone and joint injury, which makes it ideal for seniors who are suffering from arthritis or back pains. Working out in water makes an individual less achy and sore after the workout. Body joints did not have any problem with maximizing its movement.

• Some would say that they experienced faster shaping and toning of muscles when doing water exercises, compared with conducting them on land. Water aerobics could help the muscles develop 12 to 14 times faster than it does when doing in land. Since water has higher density than air, it has higher resistance which is among the reasons for better muscular development and endurance

• The heart works better when doing water aerobics. Compared to activities like running or swimming, the heart rate is maintained at a lower rate.

• This is great for burning calories and losing weight. Walking for instance, when done on land can burn about 135 calories in half an hour. If performed in water, you could burn by as much as 264 calories for the 30-minute session.

• Aqua aerobics are great for those who have arthritis, osteoporosis and pregnant because the workouts are actually gentle enough for joint movements but quick enough to build muscle mass. Still, if a person has the following medical conditions, expert's advice is still important.

Even with all the benefits, water aerobics is still not perfect. Since it would require the use of facilities and equipment, water aerobics exercise tend to be more expensive. Some health insurance providers could provide coverage for the aqua aerobics as long as it is recommended by the attending physician.

CHAPTER 4- AEROBIC BREATHING

Aerobic exercises will help to increase the level of oxygen that gets supplied to various parts of the body. The body needs ample amounts of oxygen in order to function.

Aerobics is one of the ways to lose weight and reduce risks of sickness and complications as a result of obesity and being overweight. It will also improve overall health. Aerobics could help in pumping more oxygen into the blood vessels, which can increase metabolism and burn more fat and calories. Aerobics literally means oxygen. Aerobic exercises are designed to increase oxygen intake. This practice would burn fat and improve health and fitness.

According to studies, about 300,000 adult deaths in the United States can be attributed to the lack of physical activity and unhealthy eating habits. About two thirds of adults in the U.S. are overweight, while about one-third of the adult population is obese. Adults are not the only ones suffering from weight problems. Children and teens with obesity have increased for the last years because of changes in lifestyle.

Would it be possible then to lose weight just by breathing alone?

Breathing is a crucial aspect in different kinds of exercises. In fact, in yoga, breathing properly is important. Breathing exercises could even remove stress and relax the body and mind. Breathing for weight loss is practiced by several aerobic breathing programs. Each program would have its own technique and its own advice.

However, it is important to understand that there is no weight loss program or pill that could produce dramatic results overnight. Obesity and being overweight cannot be resolved by aerobic breathing alone. Of course, proper diet and exercise is still crucial to battle the pounds away. Aerobic breathing can supplement these weight loss programs to acquire better results.

Most of us would only use about 20% of our lung capacity, while 70% of toxic elimination in our body happens when we breathe. Aerobic breathing helps our body maximize its potential. By breathing properly for about 20 minutes a day, you can bring drastic results in your health.

The guiding principle is that breathing can cleanse your body. It could help in flushing out waste, toxins and other pollutants from your body. Diaphragmatic deep breathing techniques could help in reducing cellulite; improve skin tone, blood circulation, digestion and even sleep.

With aerobic breathing, all you have to do is sit up straight, exhale from the lungs and inhale through the nose. Breathing should be able to stretch the lungs to its capacity. When exhaling, make sure to force out all the air in the lungs. Hold breathing for a while and then pull your stomach in. You can do these breathing exercises about 10 to 20 times. Some would prefer doing them before proceeding with any exercise training.

Everyone wants to lose weight. But it does not mean that you should start starving yourself and become a slave to exercise machines. In the end, losing weight would still mean eating fruits, vegetables and healthy food, exercising regularly and staying or maintaining a positive outlook of life.

Whenever we are including ourselves in aerobics and weight loss programs, setting realistic goals for us to accomplish would make it easier for us and at the same time, take weight loss according to our own phase. Breathing may not be the magic beans we're looking for to look good, but it can definitely help us change into a new person.

CHAPTER 5- AEROBIC DANCE

Aerobic dancing will not only help to burn off those excess carbs but also help to burn off excess fat.

Aerobic dancing combines exercises and different forms of dances like ballet and jazz into an exercise routine. They are usually considered low-impact exercises and slower paced compared with other aerobic routines, although there are also fast-paced routines. Because of these characteristics, they are very ideal for those who need low-impact routines like the elderly, overweight and those who are pregnant.

What makes aerobic dance an interesting routine is, of course, its music. There are different types of music which can be used for different aerobic dances. There are different speed and style variations of aerobic dances. There are guidelines for aerobic music. It is usually about 120 to 124 beats per minute for step aerobics. For low-impact exercises, it is usually about 136 to 148 beats per minute. Beginners would dance or sweat it out with slower beats.

Aerobic dance could be classified into high-impact exercises, low-impact, step aerobics and water dance aerobics. High impact exercises, as its name implies, would involve intensive exercises which includes jumping actions synchronized with the music. Step aerobics uses the step bench, and the water aerobics is performed in waist-deep water.

Aside from the movements along with the music, aerobic dance is also combined with fast or aerobic breathing. This pumps more oxygen into the blood stream, rejuvenating the body. Aerobic dances are usually done from 20 to 30 minutes, practiced for three times a week. The routine is performed just like rhythmic dances, with counts essential in setting the rhythm.

Before proceeding with the routine, getting warmed-up is important. It would usually last for 10 to 15 minutes. These stretching exercises will lower risks of injury and at the same time prepare the body for any extensive movement. After the routine proper, relaxing or cooling down movements for another 5 to 15 minutes will be performed to help the heart and the muscles relax.

Aerobic dancing has many benefits even though they were done or practiced in a fun way. This kind of aerobic workout is a great way to lose weight and at the same time, tone body muscles. It would also help the body develop strength among bones who carry most the body's weight and also toughen cardiovascular muscles.

Just like other exercises, aerobic dance can increase the circulation of the blood; reduce the levels of blood sugar and cholesterol. Because aerobic dancing would include proper breathing exercises, more oxygen is circulated in the heart, lungs and blood vessels which makes the body to function better, produce higher energy and stamina. Its physical benefits would also include boosting of the immune system, preparing the body against colds, flu, etc.

Aerobic dancing is also a great way to keep stress away. This could break the stressful and monotonous routine we have at home, school or in the work place. It can even allow you to develop or practice your creativity, since you can create your own dance steps or routine. If you cannot leave the house to go to a gym, you could do the aerobic exercises at home, learn the steps and pick your own song. How fun it is to stay healthy with aerobics by swaying your hips!

Chapter 6- Aerobic Kickboxing

Since the 1960's aerobics has been a popular form of exercise and there are numerous forms of the exercise including aerobic kickboxing.

There are different types and routines in aerobics. And one of them is aerobic kickboxing. Aerobic kickboxing should not be confused with kickboxing which is a self-defense technique. With aerobic kickboxing, which is also called cardio kickboxing, you could lose about 800 calories within an hour. Aside from losing weight, cardio kickboxing is also great in building lower and upper body strength.

Aerobic kickboxing starts just like any other kind of aerobic exercise, with five to ten minutes of warm-up. After that, it would be the kicking and punching which would end up with another five minute cool-down. This aerobic exercise combines martial-arts, self-defense, boxing and music. A person who is performing this would be able to learn the basics of these parts. For example, basic boxing stance is taught. Punches like jabs and hooks, kicks like sidekicks are taught.

Kickboxing is thought to have originated from Muay Thai. But aside from the Thai boxing influences, aerobic kickboxing also uses karate skills to develop flexibility, strength and endurance in one cardiovascular exercise. Those who practice aerobic kickboxing would also testify that it was able to help them build their self-confidence, self-esteem, self-control and develop a positive attitude towards exercising and work-out.

In addition to that, it can also reduce levels of stress and increase the individual's stamina and energy. Imagine, learning self-defense and keeping your personal fitness in check in an hour or less in a day. But as great as it is, there should be considerations before practicing aerobic kickboxing.

• Your Personal Level of Fitness

Aerobic kickboxing is a high-impact aerobic routine. Those who are suffering from arthritis, tight hamstrings and inflexible back can have difficulties with this routine. And always consider getting your doctor's advice before proceeding with any kind of exercise program especially if you have an existing medical condition.

• Consider Your Level of Expertise

If it is your first time to do such workout, then you could always get a beginning class. After being familiar with it, you could start progressing into intermediate and advance levels. If working out with a CD/DVD or tape at home, then pay attention to the instructions and start and do the workout according to your own pace. There are moves like high-kicks which should be avoided by beginners. These moves would require flexibility which would be developed later on when you have already gotten used to the routine.

• Hydrate

Always drink water before, during and after the workout.

• If the CD or the class runs for more than an hour, you are not obligated to work out for the entire period. An hour of aerobic exercise is enough.

• Wear clothes that would not restrict the flow of movements while exercising. Loose-fitting clothes could be a problem sometimes.

Jana Duncan
Cardio kickboxing could still put beginners at risk of joint injury. Especially, if they would be extending or using incorrect forms and stances like overextending kicks and locking joints. Wearing weights and holding dumbbells are also not a good idea since they could also be detrimental to your joints. When performing aerobic kickboxing or any kind of aerobics, never give in to peer pressure and excise beyond your limits or fatigue.

Keep in mind that speed, flexibility and your overall performance and fitness will increase along with regular practice.

CHAPTER 7- STEP AEROBICS

After injuring a knee, Gin Miller created step aerobics after getting advice from her orthopedic doctor that it was best to use a milk crate to step up and down to strengthen the muscles.

Aerobics, developed by Dr. Kenneth Cooper in the early seventies, had become one of today's most performed exercises. Aerobics (literally "with oxygen") is basically a form of exercise to improve one's overall fitness in muscular strength, flexibility and cardiovascular health.

One of today's more popular forms of aerobics exercises is called step aerobics, introduced at the start of the 90s. The new form is an innovation of the old aerobics routine, this time having a step (a raised contraption, 6 to 8 inches high) where the aerobics performer will step on or off from time to time.

The stepping rates (it usually starts at 120 per minute) and the height of the steps (6 to 8 inches) are adjusted according to the exerciser's needs and experience. These simple step-up, step-down aerobics are as beneficial as those of more intense movements, but less damaging to the joints.

Basic Moves

The basic step involves stepping one foot first and then the other on top of the step, and stepping down on the floor using the same sequence of foot movements. There is a general agreement among aerobic enthusiasts that the "right basic" is stepping right foot up, then the left, and then stepping down to the floor with the right then the left foot.

For variations, instructors switch different moves within the sequence, like changing the "right basic" to the "left basic" without in-between moves. Usually, this is done by way of "tapping" the foot instead of shifting weights.

Another form of step is called "tap-free" or smooth step. This is done with the feet always alternating and without the confusing "taps". The "taps" can sometimes make learning difficult for new aerobics students.

The instructor usually plans beforehand when to insert a switching move that maintains the natural rhythm of moves to simulate the natural shifting of weights on both legs like in walking.

From the right basics, the instructor might insert a "knee up" (lifting a knee and during the return, switches the move to the other foot) and continue with the left basics.

Sets

Usually, a set prepared by the instructor consists of many different moves with different durations. This is executed together by the whole class and usually timed to 32 beats per set. This is done in such a way that the whole set can be switched and repeated in the other leg, mirror-like.

Basic level classes have simpler basic moves. Advanced classes sometimes incorporate dance elements like turns and stomps and whatever is in vogue.

Elements are strung together in two to three routines per class. One learns these routines in class, which will be performed at the end of the class. Most instructors offer several choices for every person's level of intensity or dance ability during the teaching of the routines.

Benefits

Step aerobics helps burn calories and maintain weight. The amount of calories that are burned depend on the intensity, speed and the duration of the aerobic exercises.

Step aerobics helps in endurance, prevents cardiovascular diseases, and improves gait and balance. It also provides flexibility training to enhance joints movements.

Finally, step aerobics helps maintain good mental health because the workouts are fun and enjoyable, and sessions certainly release stress. With a group session, a person's social life is enhanced as well.

CHAPTER 8- AEROBICS FOR KIDS

Exercise is great for everyone, especially the children as it helps to keep them active.

It is important to teach kids early about health and fitness. Involving them in exercise and aerobics would not only help them understand health but also help them direct their energies into movements and practices that would be productive and at the same time, beneficial in the long run.

According to studies, about 25% of children and teens do not have any "vigorous physical activity." About 14% children and teens report no physical activity like walking or cycling, every day. This can be one of the reasons why the number of children has doubled since the early 1970s. In 2000, 19% of children, 6 to 11 years old, and 17%, 12 to 19 years old, are considered overweight.

Those who are involved in physical activities, reduce the risks of developing health problems as they grow older. Exercising reduces the risks of obesity, diabetes, high blood pressure, stroke and heart disease. But making your child follow a 30 minute exercise video is no fun for your kid. There are fitness centers that have children workout program, they would include biking, swimming, walking, marching, playing games to introduce low, moderate and high impact aerobics and physical activity.

Introducing children and teens to aerobics would help them become more active and at the same time, change their outlook towards the lifestyle they will be having as they grow old. There are also fitness centers which offer exercise programs suitable for children and teens, based on their age, skill and of course, their fitness and personal condition.

There are also CDs and DVDs that mix an aerobic workout with dances and other fun ways. Teens and older children may enjoy dancing to hip-hop and modern dances. Some would also show interest in doing aerobic dances, kickboxing, yoga and Pilates. You could also help your child participate in school-organized sports and activities.

There are guidelines that should be kept in mind when involving your child in physical activity according to Centers for Disease Control and Prevention (1997) and the Council for Physical Education for Children (1998). Children should at least be physically active within 30 to 60 minutes on all or most of the days of the week. Moderate to vigorous activity a day should last for about 10 to 15 minutes. Playing games and activities like biking, walking, running, etc. should also be included in the child's activities.

To encourage physical activity, make sure to implement rules that would lead to healthier lifestyle. This would include setting time for watching television and computer games. Aside from that, make sure that your child would be eating meals not in front of the television or computer. This would promote or give time for parents to talk to children during meals.

The easiest way to teach and encourage children to exercise is to set an example. Obesity and overweight problems are not just children health concerns, alarmingly, a lot of adults also suffer from these health problems. The family exercising together helps the family build stronger and closer relationships. Aerobics would not only benefit your child, but the whole family as well.

CHAPTER 9- THE BEST TYPES OF AEROBICS

There are quite a number of forms of aerobics but there are some options that are better than others.

Since the 80s, aerobics took the world of exercise by storm. Different from high intensity workouts used by professional athletes before, aerobics is a moderate exercise that is effective in improving one's overall fitness.

After being developed by Dr. Kenneth Cooper, regular aerobics exercises and routines had been enhanced and were given innovations since its inception into the mainstream of modern life.

A big part of the appeal of aerobics on almost everybody is the fact that it is simply any moderate physical activity that can be performed continuously for a certain length of time.

This type of exercise works the body at the lower end of the target heart rate area, causing the heart and lungs to adapt and become strong.

Because of this, aerobics is known as the best cardio and weight-loss exercise routine. Most bodybuilders attest that aerobics provide a sustained calorie-burning effect not matched by any exercise.

The best aerobic exercise for burning fat and losing permanent weight will depend, of course, on the individual's fitness level. If one has low fitness levels (most often, people who are just starting out), walking or step aerobics would probably be best.

Some Recommendations

For starters, the best aerobics would include walking, running, jumping rope, ski machines, treadmills, rowers, health riders and more.

If you are just starting out or have not been working out lately, the best starter program is walking. Even if the fat-burning potential in walking is low, this is a great routine for beginners.

In time, on the advice of your trainer and doctor, you can step up your routine. Perhaps, you can later jog and increase the intensity level in your fat-burning.

Running and Cycling

Running or jogging, the logical next level after your walking is rated the best aerobic exercises by many experts. It has a high fat-burning capacity, and if done with consistency, will produce obvious results every practitioner can feel and see for themselves.

One should be on alert, though, on the danger for individuals to over-train. The name of the game is moderation, especially if you have some medical history of cardio-vascular problems. As always, consult your doctor first.

Cycling, either on a stationary bike or a real one, is another fun and excellent aerobics routine. Cross-country or mountain biking not only gives you the exercise benefits you want, but will also get you to see scenic places that can excite the mind.

Treadmills and Weights

In treadmills, you can combine walking, jogging and perform resistance training as well. The possibility of doing high intensity exercise routines in treadmills makes them very effective aids in your fat-burning goals.

This is also true with other exercise gears in the gym like rowing machines. In rowing, the whole body routines can greatly help in burning calories.

On the advice of your trainer, you may add a light weight training session to your aerobics. This might be done at least thrice a week. Weight training with aerobics is a potent combination for burning fat as well as preserving and toning your muscles.

Moderation and Consistency

In all of these, the main frame of mind of the exerciser should be consistency. Aerobics needs moderation. Anything more intense is another exercise program.

CHAPTER 10- HOW-CAN-AEROBICS-HELP-YOU-LOSE-WEIGHT

As aerobics helps to burn carbohydrates and burn fat, it is a great way to lose weight.

One of the most popular means of losing weight ever since is aerobic exercises because of its long term benefits when it comes to overall health. Although many people are living testaments to the wonders of weight loss by dieting and cutting down on important nutrients, not all of these offer certain and desirable results like aerobic exercises can.

If you are one of those who are contemplating over losing weight, then now is the time to stop entertaining the thoughts on weight loss programs or diets. It is now time to conduct a little research first on aerobic exercises to help you understand how aerobics help you lose weight and achieve can long term health benefits.

Aerobics Basics

Aerobics refer to doing an activity such as a physical exercise for a longer period of time but with lesser force and effort on the part of the one who is doing it. Simply put aerobics exercises are those that allow a person to do multi-tasking such as carrying out a conversation while doing the exercise or engaging in simple yet productive activities.

The most common forms of aerobic exercises might include simple walking, jogging, swimming and even cross country skiing. To those who cannot carry on these simple exercises religiously on their own, they can try attending aerobic classes nearby where there is an instructor to lead them.

Experts say that before you engage in any activity such as aerobic exercises please make sure that you have reviewed its requirements well. Avoid choosing activities that would not suit your health and lifestyle conditions.

Also, make sure that you have visited a registered or licensed physician first before trying on aerobic exercises and before using any weight loss product that you think might complement your activity such as food supplements, herbs, or over-the-counter medications.

What Can Be Done?

To ensure that aerobic exercises will work for you, take time off to read and understand various issues surrounding it. You can check the Internet where there are thousands of sites that will lead you into any information you want on aerobic exercise or ask a person who you know that did this before so you can ask for first hand tips and suggestions. It will also help if you:

Record your eating habits and patterns by keeping a food journal. Updating and monitoring your food and eating patterns will help you track down the reasons behind your weight gain. Asking for professional help from a registered dietitian will make the monitoring more valid.

Indulge and give in if you are craving for a specific food or dish since being not overly-restrictive with food or favorite treats can be awarding experience. By giving into these cravings you can totally avoid eating foods that are high in calories and fats.

Engage yourself in only one daily exercise such as walking—which is the easiest form of aerobic exercise—since it is recommended by most authorities to help you lose weight while keeping your body fit and healthy. Other exercises and workouts that last 30 to 60 minutes will also help you burn unwanted fats and calories.

Chapter 11- Aerobics During Pregnancy

Even pregnant moms can get exercise by doing some low impact aerobic exercises.

Everybody can benefit from exercise, even those who are handicapped. The elderly would exhibit health improvements when performing low-impact exercises. Pregnant women would also benefit from low-impact aerobic exercises. Those who practice aerobics while pregnant would experience easier labor and child-birth.

There are also studies that showed women who have been performing aerobic exercises have reduced risk of undergoing caesarean operation/ surgery, quicker recovery whether it is physical or from postpartum depression. These women would also shed pounds gained during pregnancy, faster. Overall, women would testify that they had healthier pregnancy compared with other women.

Exercising while pregnant does not mean that soon-to-be-mothers would carry on the same pace or exercises they were doing prior to pregnancy. Since expecting mothers are practically sustaining two lives in their bodies, they should not be exerting too much in their exercises. Pregnant women are recommended to perform aerobic exercises for not more than 30 minutes. When exercising too much, the body temperature of both mother and child could increase. This could cause problems with the baby; excessive heat during the first trimester could cause birth defects. While later on during second trimester, it could trigger premature birth.

To avoid hyperthermia or excessive heat, exercises can be performed early in the morning when the weather is cooler. Pregnant women should drink plenty of water and avoid exerting too much force or energy, like weightlifting. Places like saunas and steam rooms should be avoided. As all pregnant women know, exercises which would make the abdomen and the stomach vulnerable should be avoided by all means. Jumping movements should also be avoided.

Light weight-lifting can also be practiced by pregnant women. This would be able to prepare them for carrying the baby after birth. Although, experts would always recommend that before proceeding to any kind of aerobic routine or program, doctor's advice is very important. Other forms of exercise which could be carried out during the first trimester would include swimming, walking, and there are special aerobic programs designed for pregnant women. While exercising, it is important to keep eat and keep your body hydrated.

During the second and last trimester, the weight of the baby could have an effect on your movements. Maintaining your balance is hard since the weight could provide stress in your joints. During this time, marching in place could replace your usual exercise routine. Exercises which would require you to bend over, spin and quick turning movements can cause the mother to lose balance and result into injury.

Use caution as you move across the floor. You may want to try a prenatal water aerobics class if one is offered in your community. It offers many of the same benefits as aerobics on land- a workout for your heart and body and the camaraderie of other expectant mothers without the stress on your joints or the risk of injury or a fall.

Jana Duncan

Even though aerobics has many benefits, doctors may not recommend it to some pregnant moms especially if they show signs of preeclampsia or worsening hypertension. The American College of Obstetricians and Gynecologists (ACOG) also cautions pregnant women against aerobic exercises that would require them to lie on their backs when they're about 20 weeks pregnant. Generally, if a pregnant woman is experiencing unusual symptoms like pain, bleeding, rapid heartbeat or dizziness, exercises should be stopped.

CHAPTER 12- AEROBIC EQUIPMENT

Aerobic equipment is not hard to get and is pretty easy to use.

Aerobics is not only good for your body but also for your overall health. It is also a great way of losing weight and keeping the unwanted pounds away. Although aerobic exercises are good as it is like kickboxing, walking, jogging or similar routines, using aerobic equipment would make exercising more fun and at the same time burn calories faster.

There are different kinds of equipment which could be used for different aerobic exercises.

• Step Bench

This is the most common equipment. The height of the step depends on the leg movements that would be used. Of course, the height would depend on the experience and expertise of the person using it. Usually, a beginner would start with a 4-inch step. As the person becomes more experienced, the height would increase to build more endurance and flexibility. One thing great about aerobic steps is that it is portable enough to be carried anywhere.

When buying a step bench, a bench with a non-slip surface will be a good idea since it would more safe. Just keep in mind that a higher step bench would mean a more intense workout.

• Stationary Bicycle

Unlike ordinary bicycles there are located only in one place. To measure the progress of the bike, an ergometer is installed. There are even stationary bikes which have computers that contain the exercise data and sessions. These bikes have different features which influence the costs of the equipment. There are different kinds of stationary bikes, buying one does not mean you would have to pick the most sophisticated and expensive model. The needs of the user come first.

• Treadmill

Treadmills can be expensive. There are manual and motorized treadmills which can be bought from different fitness centers. There are different features included in a treadmill like the pulse monitor, bottle holder, and book rack. There are even sophisticated models which would allow you to use video and audio players to kill boredom while doing the exercises. When buying treadmill, the size is the most important factor. Check if it would be able to fit into your exercise or living room area.

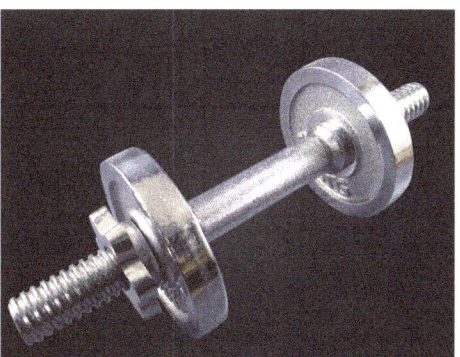

• Hand Weights

Lifting weights is another component of aerobic exercises. When seriously trying to build muscles, then start getting 3 lbs. and 5 lbs. weights. When using hand weights, users are recommended to use aerobic gloves to grip better. Water aerobics also have customized weights which can be used in aquatic exercises.

Whenever performing aerobic exercises, using the proper gear is important, the right clothes and shoes. Make sure that the clothes will allow the body to move easily, the shoes should be comfortable enough and keep the user balanced.

Aside from paying attention to wearing the proper working-out clothes, asking your doctor or health-care provider about any kind of recommendation with what kind of fitness equipment and program would be suitable for your needs is important. If buying fitness equipment is out of the option, then you could always sign-up for a membership in fitness centers, as long as they offer the equipment you would prefer to use.

Chapter 13- The Beauty Of Aerobic Exercises

If the aim is to lose weight and improve one's overall health and wellness, it is best to do some form of aerobic exercise.

Today, more and more remedies are being offered in the market for those people who would want to lose weight. Among these are weight loss remedies come in the form of products, supplements, and programs. But if there is one thing that experts would consider the safest, it would be aerobic exercises.

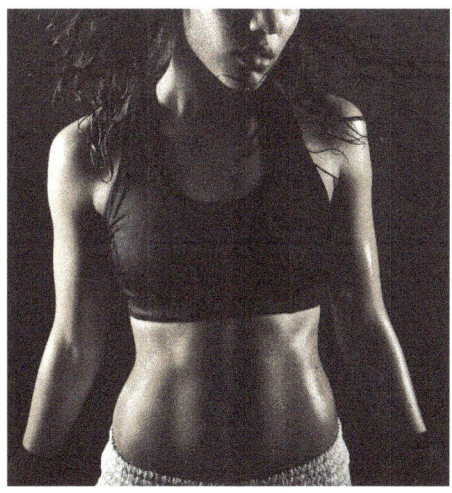

Before you engage in any weight loss diet, product, or program, make sure that you have full comprehension of its effects and possible side effects to avoid going back to your form after you lose weight. Being knowledgeable about these products and the possible risks associated with it can give you an idea what are the products you can take in, diets you can engage in or programs you can enroll with.

Most studies show that diets that promote weight loss of more than two pounds weekly are not safe because it increases the possibility of serious health problems compared to gradual weight loss. Medical experts also agree that losing weight at a slower rate may reduce risks of health problems that are closely associated with rapid weight loss.

Also, fad diets and quick weight loss products available today do not only ignore but totally violates the basic principles of good nutrition and various dietary guidelines. Do not be overwhelmed with the promise of quick weight loss because any claims that a person can lose weight almost effortlessly are fabricated.

These are just some of the reasons why more and more experts recommend safe means of cutting down on weight such as aerobics. Since aerobic exercises entail doing a lesser effort in an activity for a longer period of time, many say that this could be an effective tool to achieve long term health benefits.

How to Keep It Up

Aside serious health risks and psychological impacts brought by futile dieting, improper weight loss through the use of non-prescribed weight loss products or diets that are not proven to be effective can bring depression plus a weakened immune system. This is why experts strongly recommend safe means of being fit and slim through aerobic exercises.

Many say that losing weight can be frustrating but a rewarding feat once you have achieved your ideal weight and figure. To help you keep up the weight that you have lost in simple aerobic exercises, here are some things that you need to debunk:

- "Low Carb Diet" is the only way for you to lose weight. This is probably one of the biggest lies being promoted by the people of weight loss industry today since by cutting out all carbo and starches will only result to lack of nutrition needed by the body especially by the muscle tissues; and

- A lot of time is needed to work a weight loss program into your schedule. If you think that you cannot handle your weight loss all by yourself, then opt enrolling in a safe and responsible weight loss option such as aerobic classes that can fit into your schedule then you can even do other things for yourself.

CHAPTER 14- THE NEED FOR AEROBICS

Aerobic exercise helps reduce the onset of certain diseases like stroke, type 2 diabetes and cardiovascular disease.

Aerobics had been a worldwide phenomenon since the 80s, and most of the world knows about it. For the uninitiated, Dr. Kenneth Cooper (its developer) submitted the official definition to the Oxford English Dictionary.

Accordingly, aerobics is defined as "a method of physical exercise for producing beneficial changes in the respiratory and circulatory systems by activities which require meeting a modest increase of oxygen intake and so can be maintained."

Because of today's many new illnesses (hypertension, type 2 diabetes, and other cardiovascular conditions) brought about by modern man's generally inactive physical lifestyle, experts strongly recommend aerobics for everyone.

Aerobic Exercise

The common definition of aerobics is simply the activity that consists of low-intensity repetitive motions of mostly the large muscles of the arms and legs for a period of time. This activity increases breathing and heart rate.

Most low-intensity activities you do during the day also fall under this category. It includes such regular activities as walking, jogging, swimming, and cycling.

For individuals who are beginners in exercise programs, or maybe have histories of health conditions, light exercise routines are recommended at first on most days of the week.

Cardiovascular Benefits

Experts advise that these aerobic exercises have to be performed at moderate intensity. This level of activity is safe for almost everyone, and it still provides the desired health benefits.

Recent research brings in additional good news. It is revealed that aerobics performers can still have cardiovascular benefits even if the exercise routine (usually 30 minutes total) is broken into three or four 8-10 minute segments, as long as they are of the same intensity.

Intensity

Doctors, however, discourage infrequent bouts of high-intensity aerobics routines. It is found that this approach is not very healthy.

In the first place, reduction in risks of hypertension, high cholesterol, type 2 diabetes and other conditions depends on the total volume of the exercise done, rather than on intensity.

Higher intensity exercise activities raise your chances for muscle or joint injury. Worse, it may trigger fatal consequences because of heart rhythm disturbances.

Aerobics instructors always begin their sessions with light stretching and low-intensity movements for about 5 to 10 minutes. This warm-up routine is important to avoid injury. At the end of the routine, a similar cooling-down period for about 5 to 10 minutes is also done.

Benefits

As had been proven these years, people who engaged in regular aerobics have been known to benefit by way of lower blood cholesterol counts, lower blood pressure, toned body because of fat reduction and beneficial weight loss.

They have been known to have developed muscular and overall body endurance, have a happier disposition and moods, and a medically-certified general lower risk to cardiovascular diseases.

Common Activities

The best part is the easy way on how to do your aerobics, even without going to the gym and participating in gym routines.

Doctors recommend a simple walk that totals around 10,000 steps a day. Start with something lower, and add the number of steps slowly every day until you reach your goal.

Done on a regular basis, brisk walking is guaranteed to erase your common health risks. Your need for aerobics is not be that hard to fill up.

About The Author

I'm passionate about working out and coming up with new workout routines; especially for aerobics as it's such a full-body workout and so good for you. I've been doing this for quite some years and don't see myself stopping any time soon. It truly has been a way of life for me. Although I have an extremely busy schedule, I find a way to get it done.

A lot of what I encourage in my books is how to set exercise goals that you can be comfortable with and actually achieve without getting too flustered. There is something that can be designed for everyone depending on their specific needs. I've found mine and helping others to find theirs is what I set out to do.

My children are teenagers now and although I put no pressure on them to work out as I do, I set an example and am pleased to see how much they respect what I do and how they are so much more conscientious of their health as they continue to develop.

www.ingramcontent.com/pod-product-compliance
Lightning Source LLC
Chambersburg PA
CBHW071143280526
45787CB00003B/1393